Intermittent Fasting

The Complete Beginner's Guide to Lose Weight Fast, Gain Energy & Live Healthy.

Intermittent Fasting and Ketogenic diet

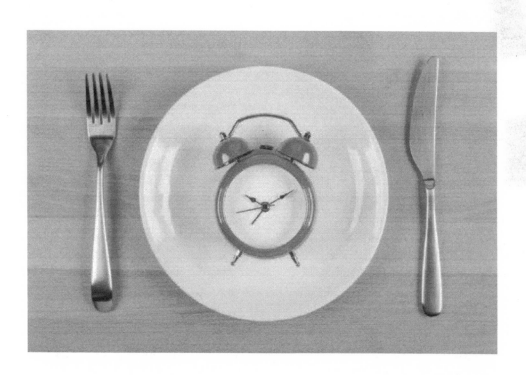

Brandon Hearn © 2018

Table of Contents

An Introduction to Intermittent Fasting

Intermittent fasting, I exactly what it sounds like. It's where someone uses a normal diet when they're eating, and they alternate with periods where they have restricted eating. It's a pattern of skipping meals, and it's something that is used on a regular basis by many people. However, restricted eating can mean anything from zero calories to a very small quantity of food that has minimized your calorie intake.

A lot of people find that intermittent fating is an effective weight loss plan. The hunger pangs can be hard to ignore, and you'll need to watch the clock. However, after you adjust your schedule, it becomes easier to handle and you get into a daily groove. It allows you to focus on when you can eat instead of what you can eat. You just have to make sure you don't overcompensate by binging between fats.

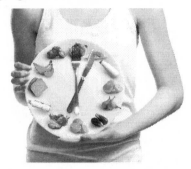

Intermittent fasting isn't right for everyone, but it does come with a variety of health benefits which will be explored later in life. If you've ever suffered from an eating disorder, then it isn't recommended that you use intermittent fasting as a weight loss deal. Before you decide if intermittent fasting is for you, you also need to consult with your doctor. If you are on any prescription medication that you have to take on a regular basis, then fasting may not work for you. Many prescription medications need to be taken with food, which will break your fast and keep you from reaping the benefits of this meal plan.

If you wish to commit to intermittent fasting, you should view it as a lifestyle change. If you view it with a casual attitude, then it likely won't work out for you. Your social life will also be a factor. You won't be able to casually go out eating or drinking with friends and family. If you start to obsess over food the moment you start to feel hunger pangs, then this diet may make you miserable, so it should be avoided. Though, for most people there is some form of intermittent fasting that will fit their lifestyle and their needs.

Common Myths

No matter what diet you take, you'll get some naysayers or people that want to interject their opinion. That's why it's best to know the facts before you begin. You'll find some common myth below.

- **It's Starvation:** You'll feel hungry at first, and some people will even say they're starving, but this isn't the case. Starvation is when you don't have sufficient food with no prospects for food in the future. It's a starvation of calories without a choice. When you're fasting, you're choosing to restrict your calories. At the end of the fast, you'll be able to get food. It won't make you move into starvation mode to fast either. Your body only shuts down the metabolism when you alter your calorie consumption drastically. There is evidence that proves that fasting for up for forty-eight hours can speed up your metabolism because of an increase in hormones. Just don't fast for more than forty-eight hours or your metabolism will slow down. Intermittent fasting is all about timing.

- **You Need Small Meals:** This isn't true either. Many people have gotten comfortable with the idea that you need three to six small meals a day, but this isn't the case. It's all about the number of calories you take in every day. It doesn't matter the amount of meals you eat. You'll only burn ten percent of your calorie consumption on digesting food. That's what the habits you have are more important than the meals you eat. Frequent small meals will only help to stave off hunger pangs, but they don't do anything for your actual health.

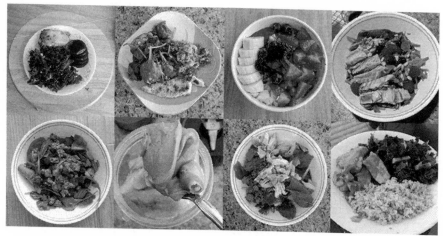

- **Your Brain Won't Get Glucose:** Many people are misguided in the belief that your brain will be deprived of glucose when you fast, but once again it just isn't true. Your brain does need glucose, but your brain can run on something other than glucose and be just fine. When your brain can't get glucose due to prolonged periods without eating, which is fasting, then your body turns to ketone bodies that are produced as fatty acids are burned. They're a great fuel for the brain.

- **You'll Lose Muscle:** Your body funs out of fuel after a month or more, which means it'll start to break down muscle. However, that is a whole month or so without food. This isn't going to happen just because you use intermittent fasting. Your body will only consume fat as a last resort. Intermittent fasting is safe to anyone in good health for up to four days, but it is not recommended to fast over forty-eight hours.

- **You'll Gain Weight:** If you do intermittent fasting properly, you won't gain weight. This is only true if you overeat when you aren't fasting. It all depends on your individual behavior. You just need to get used to the fasting, and your appetite may even diminish as you continue with it. Non-fasting calories just need to stay below the calories missed while fasting for you to lose weight.

- **It'll Hurt Your Health:** A lot of people believe that when you fast you deprive your body of nutrients that it needs to stay health, but once again it's far from true. It's been proven that intermittent fasting has a variety of health benefits, which will be discussed later in this book.

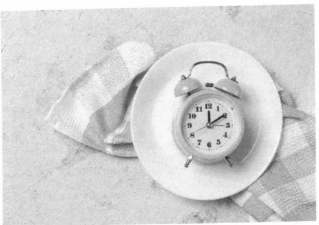

Different Intermittent Fasting Methods

There are a few different ways that you can approach intermittent fasting. Just chose the method that works best for you.

16:8 Method

This is a time restricted fasting method. It's appealing to people who find it impossible to go a full day or more without food. In this method, you'll generally fast for sixteen hours, and then you'll eat high quality foods for the remaining eight hours. It can be modified to the 12/12 or 20/4 method as well. Some people do use other combinations, but the 16/8 is the recommended. Simply skipping one meal a day can do the trick for most people! You must sleep for six to eight hours anyways, which will count towards part of your last.

Those hours can be subtracted from active fasting time. While you don't have to limit the amount of meals you have during your non-fasting time, you should try to eat wholesome food. Try to avoid junk food, and make sure that you don't over eat in anticipation to the fasting period. You should have a planned workout during the day, and it's okay to eat healthy carbs on days you're working out.

Just try to cut back on your meals when you don't have a workout that day. During your fasting period remember to drink plenty of water, especially since you won't be eating anything. It's best to drink water, but you can also have black coffee, hot or iced tea, and other no-calorie beverages. Staying hydrated can also help to lessen your hunger pangs.

Below you'll find a sample schedule of this intermittent fasting method based on someone getting up at 7 a.m. and going to bed 11 p.m. to get eight full hours of sleep. In this example, you're choosing to skip your meals in the morning instead of later in the evening, so your first eight hours of fasting has been from 11 p.m. the night before to 7 a.m. when you wake up. You still need to go eight more hours before eating.

7 a.m.	Wake Up	Remember to Stay Hydrated
3 p.m.	First Meal	A healthy "breakfast" could include whole wheat pancakes, a drink of your choice, sausage or bacon, and a boiled egg.
5 p.m.	Snack Time	You will want to eat a piece of fruit, cheese and crackers, or raw vegetables
7 p.m.	Second Meal	For your second meal most people prefer to go with something that's more "dinner" time. This could include baked chicken, steamed broccoli, and a baked potato. You can even have a dinner roll!
9 p.m.	Snack Time	A healthy dessert is recommended, but any dessert within moderation is acceptable.
11 p.m.	Go to Bed	This starts the beginning of your next fast

Eat Stop Eat Method

This is a 24-hour fast method, and it should only be used once or twice a week. You eat dinner on day one, then you would restrict yourself from having any food until dinner time on the second day. However, it can be modified where you eat breakfast to lunch instead, but you'll still fast for twenty-four hours at a time. You'll then resume a normal eating pattern until your next "stop" day where you do this again.

You can have one to two "stop" days a week. With this method you don't need to count calories, fats or carbs. Within reason you can even indulge in a sweet treat every now and then. By cutting down the hours you're eating, it'll help to reduce the overall calories you take in. even if you over indulge every once in a while, it'll be hard to replace the calories missed from an entire twenty-four hours of fasting.

However, with this method you will want to focus on weight training to ensure your muscle integrity. It's also designed to be flexible, so if twenty-four hours is too long at first, you can start with eight hours, and then the next stop day can be twelve hours, and you'll keep moving it up until you can go twenty-four hours without eating.

You'll find an example schedule below based on this method.

Sunday	7 a.m. Wake Up	You Can Eat	6 p.m. Dinner No Snacking	11 p.m. Bed
Monday	7 a.m. Wake Up	Don't Eat	6 p.m. Dinner	11 p.m. Bed
Tuesday	7 a.m. Wake Up	You Can Eat	6 p.m. Dinner	11 p.m. Bed
Wednesday	7 a.m. Wake Up	You Can Eat	6 p.m. Dinner	11 p.m. Bed
Thursday	7 a.m. Wake Up	You Can Eat	6 p.m. Dinner	11 p.m. Bed
Friday	7 a.m. Wake Up	Don't Eat	6 p.m. Dinner No Snacking	11 p.m. Bed
Saturday	7 a.m. Wake Up	You Can Eat	6 p.m. Dinner	11 p.m. Bed

Below you'll find an example meal plan for one of the days you can eat on this method.

7 a.m. Wake Up	When you wake up, it's best to wait until breakfast at 10 a.m. However, you can have crackers or an apple to start your metabolism.
10 a.m.	You should indulge in a healthy breakfast such as Greek yogurt, fresh fruit, and granola to get your day started.
1 p.m.	You can have a healthy lunch such as a tuna salad sandwich with raw carrots and dip. Almost any salad with light dressing would also be a healthy option.
3 p.m.	It's okay to have a healthy snack such as a fat bomb if you're on the keto diet or a piece of fruit or raw vegetables for others.
6 p.m.	This is a great time for dinner, and a healthy, lean protein, steamed or pan seared vegetable, and small starch such as sweet potato or brown rice is a great choice.
8:30 p.m.	This is the latest that you should have a snack if you're going to bed at 11. If you're having something sweet, keep it small, and make sure it has as little sugar or carbs as possible. A poached pear is a wonderful sweet treat that's still a relatively healthy choice.
11 p.m. Bed Time	Do not Snack.

The 5:2 Method

If you have a hard time going without food, then you'd want to try this modified fasting method. It's a weekly cycle where you have two days that are non-consecutive where you'll reduce your normal intake of calories to only twenty-five percent of your normal calorie consumption. For women, you'll want to stick to about 500 calories, and men will want to stick to about 600 calories. You can choose to consume them in one sitting or you can spread them out throughout the day. One the other five days, you'll want to follow a healthy, normal diet. When you reach your desired weight, you'll likely want to modify this diet to only one day out of every six instead of two out of every seven.

It'll help to keep you from losing too much weight, and you can always go back to the 5:2 method when you want to lose the weight again. This may be the case after holiday splurging for example. Remember that it's best to eat wholesome foods, and don't overeat. You may not feel satisfied on fasting days, but it should help to calm your hunger pangs by eating healthy foods with lower calories.

With this diet, just use good judgement. Just follow what's best for you and make informed choices. High fiber and high protein foods are the best things to eat on a fasting day so that you can feel full on lower calories. Some great choices are fish, lean meat, vegetables, eggs, yogurt, berries and soups. You will also need to stay hydrated. So, drink plenty of water, and you can enjoy zero calorie beverages, green tea, and black tea, black coffee and herbal tea as desired.

Below you'll find an example of a fasting day for women. If you're a man, then choose something that has 100 more calories. Remember that we're going on an example schedule where you wake up at 7 a.m. and go to bed at 11 p.m.

7 a.m.	A spinach omelet will come to roughly 90-100 calories
12 p.m.	You can have chicken miso soup for a low-calorie filling lunch will roughly be about 130-150 calories depending on your recipe. You can find any soups within this range.
4 p.m.	You can get a Chinese vegetable chow mein for roughly 180-200 calories depending on your recipe.
9 p.m.	This allows for a 30-50 calorie snack, such as a single egg or even a piece of fruit. Just be careful what type of fruit you get! Carrot sticks are also a healthy option.

Up Day Down Day Fasting

This is also known as alternate day fasting. This is one day fasting and one day feeding, and you repeat it like you would in the 5:2 method, but it has a 4:3 program. People who practice this method are likely to lose an average of three to eight percent of their body weight within about twenty-four weeks. It should result in no decreases in your metabolism. Below you'll find a week-long schedule of when to eat and when not to eat using this method.

Sunday	Eat Normally
Monday	Restrict Your Calories
Tuesday	Eat Normally
Wednesday	Restrict Your Calories
Thursday	Eat Normally

Friday	Restrict Your Calories
Saturday	Eat Normally

Below you'll find another example of a 500-calorie diet, which you'll use on restricted calorie days. Remember that if you stay hydrated, you're less likely to feel hunger pangs as severely during your restricted days.

7 a.m.	Almonds, a small amount of granola and Greek yogurt will come to about 100 to 120 calories.
12 p.m.	A small salad will come to about 170-200 calories. Just remember that dressing will be the biggest calorie factor.
4 p.m.	A Vegetable over couscous can come to about 200-250 calories depending on your recipe.
9 p.m.	Remember that fresh vegetables or a piece of fruit is a great way to have a small snack before bed. Two small satsumas are usually under 50 calories.

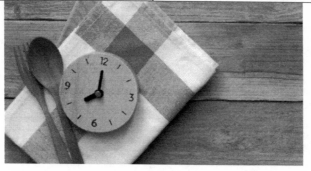

Benefits of Intermittent Fasting

When you fast, you'll need to adapt to the situation, you'll notice that there are a range of benefits to intermittent fasting. Your body has a natural defense mechanism to a lack of nourishment which makes it create different enzymes and hormones which benefit you. '

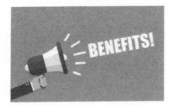

You'll Lose Weight

When you eat fewer meals, you consume fewer calories. So long as you don't overcompensate by consuming too many calories when you aren't fasting, then you'll lose weight. With the hormonal changes your body will also experience an enhanced metabolic function which can contribute to weight loss. In most cases, when intermittent fasting issued properly, you won't need to count calories. When your body has adapted to eating three meals a day, your body stores the food as glucose for energy. It can take your body ten to twelve hours to use up a single supply of glucose from a single meal. With a constant supply of food to store as glucose, the body doesn't see a need to turn to the stored fat as an energy source.

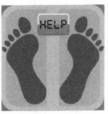

A Reboot of Hormones

Even when you're not eating, your body doesn't rest and do nothing. When you start fasting, your pancreas will take a break from producing insulin. However, the pituitary gland starts to produce extra human growth hormone (HGH). If you're an adult, then you've already stopped growing, but this hormone is still important for cell regeneration. The hunger hormone ghrelin has been shown to be affected positively by intermittent fasting. The changes in ghrelin releases will improve dopamine levels in the brain, which will also improve cognitive function by regulating these hormones and chemicals.

Reduced Free Radicals

Free radicals are unstable, so they'll attack your other molecule including enzyme, proteins and your DNA which cause damage. They also produce toxins that can help you to fight infection and inflammation. However, an overproduction of free radicals will cause inflammation another harmful effects such as a higher risk of stroke, rheumatoid arthritis, ulcers, dementia, premature aging of your skin, and much more. It's one reason that a hormone reboot is vital to helping stave off the effects of aging and get your body functioning optimally.

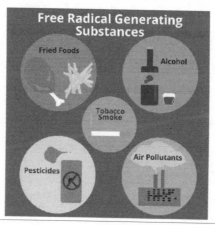

Better Brain Function

You already know that reduced blood sugar levels, lower inflammation, and a reduction of oxidative stress is beneficial to your body, but it's great for your brain too. Brain Derived Neurotropic Factor is a protein in the brain that impacts the function of the peripheral nervous system and the brain itself. Fasting will increase this protein, which will help your brain to grow and develop further. It can help with loss of memory, diminished cognitive ability, and it can even help to fight depression.

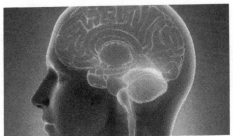

Lower Risk of Cardiovascular Disease

Heart disease is the leading cause of death for men and women. Your lifestyle habits can reduce the risk of cardiovascular disease and choosing to intermittently fast will help as well. Intermittent fasting will lower blood sugar levels, lower blood pressure, lower insulin levels, and lower LDL and total cholesterol. It'll even lower your triglycerides and decrease overall inflammation in the body, which all helps with cardiovascular health.

A Longer Lifespan

There are many studies that indicate that intermittent fasting can slow down the aging process. It can also help to fight off age related diseases. Your body believes fasting to be a situation of stress, so your cells will adapt to deal with it. So, a result, your body can cope with stress better, and therefore can deal with stressors such as disease a little easier.

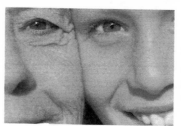

Reduced Risk of Diabetes

When people are overweight or obese, they have a higher chance of developing type 2 diabetes. Many people have been diagnosed weigh prediabetes, which is a wakeup call to start a healthier lifestyle before they become a diabetes 2 statistic. Intermittent fasting helps to lower insulin resistance so that your blood sugar levels can drop. Losing weight will increase your insulin sensitivity, which will help to keep your blood sugar stable as well.

An Improved Digestive System

When you fast, you allow your digestive system to time to rest, repair and revitalize itself. When you aren't eating all the time, then your body isn't going to need to digest anything. That allows your digestive organs time to eliminate toxins and waste from the body.

Intermittent Fasting & Cancer

Intermittent fasting is a great way to help decrease your risk of getting many types of cancers, but it is also recommended to cancer patients to help them. However, you'll need to talk to your doctor to make sure that it's right for you. In this chapter, we'll explore why it's recommended for cancer patients and how it can help to decrease your chance of developing certain cancers.

For Cancer Patients

Intermittent fasting is recommended for some cancer patients because it can help to trigger the immune system to fight cancer. Your immune system has a hard time finding, targeting and killing your body's abnormal cells, which are cancer cells. There are various cancer treatments that re being developed to stimulate the immune system to do this. With the fasting diet along with chemotherapy, the immune system has been proven to target and kill cancer cells better, including the B and T cells, which can help to target and kill tumor cells.

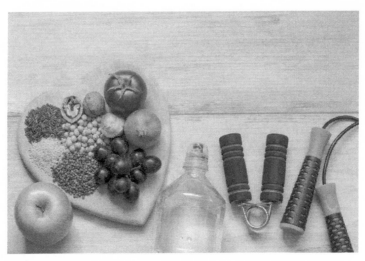

It's believed that this helps the chemotherapy drugs to work better. The same research was conducted through human cancer patients as well, and it can slow tumor growth in cancer patients. It's also been proven to help reduce cancer recurrence and mortality rates. Fasting may also help to reduce the side effects that are a result of cancer treatment, especially chemotherapy. These side effects can range from debilitating or uncomfortable. Patients that have participated I the fasting diet have experienced less weakness, fewer headaches, less fatigue, no vomiting and less nausea in the studies up until this point. It has also helped some patients with mouths ores, dry mouth, cramps and numbness.

Cancer Prevention

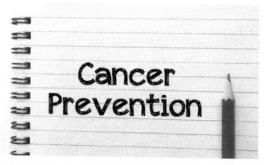

So far, the research that intermittent fasting can help to prevent cancer has only been proven in animals. However, it has had good enough results to warrant human study. Since intermittent fasting helps with your blood sugar levels, hormone levels, helps to rest your body, decreases obesity, and helps cell regeneration, it can severely lower your risk of cancer.

Fasting & Muscle Gain

If you want to gain muscle, you may be hesitant to try intermittent fasting, but you shouldn't worry. The formula for gaining muscle is the same formula at first as gaining fat. Your calorie consumption should include protein if you wish to build muscle. Fasting isn't the most effective way to gain muscle, but it's a great to make sure that you aren't gaining fat while you tone down and build the diet and target weight you need to start toning your muscle and gaining it properly.

If you wish to gain muscle while using intermittent fasting, then you'll need to add in weight and resistance training as well to your schedule. However, without some form of exercise, you will not be able to retain or even build muscle mass during intermittent fating. The recommended amount of protein is 0.8 grams per pound of body weight when you're trying to maintain muscle. If you're trying to build muscle, then it's even more important to increase that amount of protein.

However, do not eat only protein, or you will be deriving your body of the essential nutrients that it needs. Therefore, it's best to use a restricted calorie intake fast, such as the 5:2 fast if you wish to use it while also building muscle mass. This way you can concentrate on protein and fiber during your restricted calories days, so that you're still supplying your body with the building blocks to get the protein you need.

However, when you're pairing weight loss with trying to build muscle mass, the weight loss will slow. This doesn't mean you aren't losing fat. It's important to keep in mind that muscle weighs more than fat, so if your fat is being replaced by muscle, you may end up weighing more. It's easier to see how many inches you are losing and to evaluate how tone you are getting instead of just counting your progress by the pounds.

Fasting Tips & Tricks

Intermittent fasting has various proven health benefits, but it can be tricky if you haven't done it before. That's where these tips and tricks can come in handy.

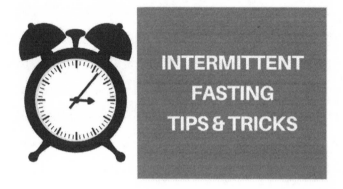

Don't Fast in Stressful Situations

Fasting is a lot of stress on your body, and that's the point. Fasting is meant to provoke a stress response from your body so that you can reap the benefits. In the case of mental stress, it'll increase your cravings for food, especially sweets, so it'll be harder to fast in stressful situations. If you are dealing with a particularly stressful situation, such as a family emergency, then it's best to take a break from your fasting diet and then resume as soon as possible. There's no reason to set yourself up for failure or cause more stress in a situation that you can't get out of.

Work Out Slowly

If you aren't used to fasting, you may not be able to work out on fasting days without allowing your body time to adjust first. This means you may only feel up to taking a short walk for the first few weeks that you get used to your fasting diet. Instead, you should concentrate on working out on your non-fasting days. You should also make sure that you don't overdo your workouts, even when you are used to fasting.

If you overdo it, then you're more likely to want to over divulge in food. If you already are used to intensive workouts, that doesn't mean it's safe to use intermittent fasting with this workouts. For example, if you're a fan of CrossFit and already participate, you may still want to take some time off from CrossFit when you begin to change over to the intermittent fasting lifestyle. That doesn't mean that you can't take CrossFit back up later.

Use Herbs & Spices

If you're using an intermittent fasting method that allows for calorie intake even when fasting, then you'll want to use herbs and spices. This will help you to flavor your food easily without adding excessive calories like butter, sauces, or salad dressing will. This means you won't sacrifice taste just to get full.

Sleep is Important

Not only is sleep important to regulate your overall health, including your hormones, but it really does help with intermittent fasting. While you don't want to sleep the day away, try to get a full eight hours of sleep a night. Sleep does count towards your fast, and you're much more likely to be able to get through a twelve to sixteen hour fast if eight of it was spent asleep in your bed.

Caffeine is a Friend

While you don't want to rely on caffeine permanently, caffeine is your friend in the beginning of intermittent fasting. You'll want to drink black coffee or black tea to help get you the caffeine you need to help blunt your appetite and keep you going even as your body starts to adjust. Just remember not to overdo it or you may feel nauseous or even jittery, which will make it hard to continue. Remember that everything should be done in moderation.

Don't Just Eat Salad

A lot of people assume that since salads are high in fiber and low in calories that they can get away with just eating salad during their calorie restricted fasts. This may seem like a good idea on paper, but it can be harmful. Remember that you need a variety of nutrients and minerals, and you'll need protein to continue to build muscle or at least not lose the muscle you have. If you are going to give in and eat a salad, make sure that it's one that's rich in protein as well as foods that are dense in nutrients and high in fiber. You may want to consider adding flaxseeds and grilled chicken to your salads for example.

Maintain a Disciplined Diet

The cravings for food increases as you fast, and it's completely natural. When you stop fasting, you'll want to over indulge. It' important to maintain discipline when you're on a "Feeding" day. You can't look at a non-fasting day as a free day to indulge on just about anything you want. This is an incorrect method to follow the routine.

Excess eating or eating very rich food will only make your fasting days more difficult. If you indulge in processed food with artificial sweeteners, then it'll be even harder to stick to a discipline. You'll also need to make sure that you don't over eat just because you can eat or you'll stretch your stomach back out again instead of allowing for your stomach to naturally shrink due to your fasting schedule.

Always Keep Hydrated

This has been stated before in this book, but it can't be stressed enough just how important it is to stay hydrated, especially during fasting days. If you are hydrated, you're less likely to feel hunger pangs. It can also help to curb cravings. Green tea has been known to help with sugar cravings, and black tea can help with caffeine withdrawals.

Don't Allow for Temptation

It's best to set up your schedule where you don't have to resist temptation all the time. You'll want to stock your kitchen with fruits and vegetables, but you'll also want to make sure that you aren't going to social events that will tempt you on your fasting days.

Always Keep an Eye on Discomfort

You should never ignore the signal that your body sends to you. If you're feeling hungry restless or tired, it's to b expected to a certain degree when fasting. However, make sure that it stays within your tolerable limits. If you are truly having a hard time with the intermittent fasting schedule you've chosen, try to gradually work your way up to it. If you feel serious signals such as dizziness, muscle weakness, or heart palpitations, then you need to consult your doctor immediately. You should not continue to fast in these situations because it can be dangerous. Do not ignore the signs of your body.

Always Exercise

Intermittent fasting is a great way to cut down fat, but that doesn't mean you shouldn't exercise. Exercise helps the weight loss process, but it also helps your general health. Make sure that you exercise at least a few times a week. It's especially important if you are hoping to tone as well as trim the excess fat.

Keep Positive

It can be hard to stick to any diet or lifestyle change if you aren't positive about it. If you have a negative outlook, you're setting yourself up for failure. That's why it's important to try to stay positive and keep away the hunger pangs so that you can stick to your diet. Remember that every day you make it is a success and count your little successes to help build momentum.

Monitor Your Progress

While it isn't important to measure only your weight loss, you may want to take pictures of your progress or at least keep a dairy of your progress. When you can look back and see your success, you're more likely to be able to continue forward with intermittent fasting easier because you don't feel discouraged. It allows you to maintain your positivity and build on the momentum that each new success brings. By taking pictures of your progress, you can visually compare yourself as you move forward with an intermittent fasting lifestyle.

Use a Buddy System

It can be helpful to stay positive and stick to a new lifestyle change if you aren't doing it alone. It'll be harder for you if you live in a household with other people and you're the only person that's trying to commit to intermittent fasting. If you have a partner, see if they'll take this journey with you. Just remember that children should not try intermittent fasting since they are still growing, and unless you've consulted with their doctor, they should stick to a normal eating schedule. By having a pattern, it'll be easier to hold yourself accountable, and you'll be able to tell each other if you see the other slipping. Sometimes we make mistakes, and you shouldn't beat yourself up over them. When you make a mistake, just try to redirect yourself back to the intermittent fasting lifestyle, and remember not to get discouraged. Being negative will only make it harder, so concentrate on what you can do to improve instead of what you've done wrong.

Controlling Your Hunger

Controlling your hunger can be an issue, but with the tips in this chapter, it'll become much easier. You already know the basic tip which is to stay hydrated!

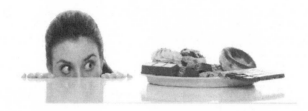

Calorie Free Beverages

It's important to consume calorie free beverages so that you don't get bored when you're trying to stay hydrated. This includes black tea, herbal tea and black coffee. It'll also help to suppress your cravings for food. These calorie free beverages will also help to reduce stress and they even have a lot of antioxidants. These beverages have detoxification properties. However, you still need to make sure to consume any beverages other than water in small quantities.

Keep Busy

If you're busy, then your mind can't focus on hunger pangs as much. Its best if you can remain engaged in work or on a personal project. This will keep your mind from straying towards food. Your metabolic rate also increases in this state, so it allows you to become more produced in your work as well. You can even tea this time to volunteer, spend more time with friends and family by inviting them to your home or pick up a hobby in nature, such as hiking or fishing.

The important thing is to keep your mind busy and your body away from the temptations of fast food or your fridge. Spending time outside of the house is only helpful if you're sure you can stay away from snacks and fast food. If you are unsure or if you're not an outdoors person, then you'll want to try to find a hobby indoors. It can even be binge reading your favorite book series.

Go for Walks

Physical activity will affect intermittent fasting positively. It keeps your mind from thoughts of eating, and if you're out doing something you're less compelled to give into your cravings. It'll help you to get in some mild exercise even on days you feel fatigued as well.

Meditate

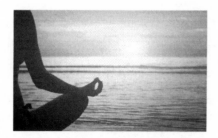

Mediation is a great way to keep your cool, and it'll help you to control your hunger and senses better. Mindfulness meditation is an easy meditation process that works great for intermittent fasting, and it can help you to stay positive during the process as well. If you stay calm, it helps to reduce the stress on you mentally even when you're causing stress on the body.

Eat Healthy

Healthy foods will help you to feel fuller for longer because it's giving your body the vitamins and nutrients that you need. It's best to carry healthy snacks with you while you're fasting as well. It'll serve two purpose. If your fasting time ends while you're out, you can eat healthy food that you already have on hand. It'll also help that if you give into temptation you'll at least only be eating a healthy choice.

Use Protein Rich Foods

Protein rich foods will help with intermittent fasting because they'll induce feelings of fullness quickly without adding too many calories. You'll need protein to build muscle mass as well. Eating lots of fresh vegetable sand fruits will also help you to stay full.

Lifestyle Hacks

Remember that intermittent fasting is a lifestyle choice, so it's important to use these lifestyle hacks if you want to be successful. You already know fasting tips and tricks and ways to control your hunger, but these hacks concentrate on a healthy lifestyle to add in on non-fasting days.

Hack #1 Toss the Junk

It's important that you toss the junk food if you want to be successful. While you can afford to indulge occasionally, remember that every calorie count. You don't want to waste calories by consuming empty calories that provide your body with nothing, which will only take you out of ketosis.

Hack #2 Put Aside 30 Minutes

It's important to put aside a half hour a day for exercise. It doesn't matter if it's light exercise or intense exercise, depending on what your health goals are. Even if you just walk for thirty minutes a day, you'll help your health and weight loss goals along.

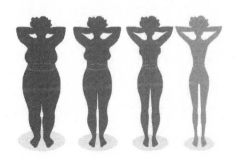

Hack #3 Set a Timer

It can help to set a timer if you've just started fasting and knowing when you can break your fast can be important. Your phone is a great way to keep track of time and set alarms to tell you when you should eat. After all, you don't want to get too busy meditating, walking, working or just enjoying yourself where you don't meet your calories goals before your fast begins.

Hack #4 Have Some You Time

Since keeping a positive outlook is important to keeping to any diet, it's important that you set aside some time just for yourself. Do what you love, and it'll help to relive stress and stave off depression, anxiety and undo stress.

Hack #5 Follow Good Nutrition

You'll learn in the coming chapter how important good nutrition is, and what good nutrition is. It's more than just voiding temptation and lowering your carb intake. You should know what foods you're putting in your body and what effect they have on you.

Hack #6 Avoid Social Events When Needed

It's important that you avoid unnecessary social events when you're busy fasting. If you go to social events when you can't eat or drink a beverage with calories, such as going to a bar with friends, you're setting yourself up for failure. If you must reschedule your fast days, then you should. However, it's easier to reschedule your social events instead, especially if you want to have an easier time sticking to your intermittent fasting in the future.

Using Good Nutrition

No matter if you're following intermittent fasting or using intermittent fasting with the keto diet, you will still need to understand what good nutrition is and how it affects your body. Good nutrition is a diet that has all the important nutrients, and it makes sure that you follow portion control. If you fail to follow good nutrition, then it'll result in nutrient deficiencies which will affect your health.

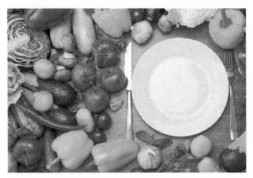

Protein

Protein is important for skin health, hair, and most importantly muscle health. It also helps with bodily reactions. Amino acids are needed for human growth, and you'll find many amino acids in protein. The best source is lentils, eggs and fish, but most meat works.

Carbs

Yes, carbohydrates are needed to some degree to follow good nutrition. When you're following the ketogenic diet, you'll limit your carbs, but you never truly cut them out. There are two types of carbs. There are simple carbs and complex carbs. Simple carbs are digested easily, and they're more likely to result in fat. You'll want to avoid simple carbs when you can, and instead choose complex carbs. Fruits and grains are sources of simple carbs, but beans and vegetables are often sources of compel carbs, which aid in digestion for example, fiber is a carb that is needed by your body.

Fats

Fats play a huge role in your health, and both polyunsaturated and monounsaturated fats are healthy. You'll find monounsaturated fats in nuts and avocados. You can find polyunsaturated fats in seafood, but of course these aren't the only places to find these healthy fats. Unhealthy fats that are not a part of good nutrition include saturated fats and Trans-fat, which you'll find mostly in junk food.

Vitamins

Vitamin A, B, C, D, E, and K are important to your body's health. A deficiency in these will only lead to healthy problems as well as a weakened immune system. If you're following good nutrition, you'll get all of the vitamins you need for your body to function.

Minerals

Minerals such as iodine calcium, iron and zinc are important to your body's health. They can be found in various foods including meats, grains and vegetables. It's not hard to get essential minerals when you're following a healthy diet.

Water

Water is important to the human body because the human body has a large amount of water in its composition. It's an essential nutrient for your body to function, which is another reason that it's essential for you to stay hydrated.

Why It's Important

The main reason that good nutrition is important is that it keeps your body functioning at optimal levels. It reduces the risk of cancer, high blood pressure, and it lowers your cholesterol. Good nutrition also increases as your immune system as well as energy.

Intermittent Fasting & the Keto Diet

There are many fans of the ketogenic diet out there, and it leaves a lot of people wondering if they can add intermittent fasting into the regimen to help further their health and weight loss goals. The keto diet already involves high amounts of fat, very low carbs, and some protein so that your body enters a state of ketosis. This diet provides people with a range of benefits, but when you add in intermittent fasting it can help to accelerate the process of autophagy which will enhance the benefits.

Since the primary goal of the keto diet is entering ketosis so that your body will burn fat instead of glucose, its' primary goal is to produce ketone bodies. When you add intermittent fasting, it allows you to get into ketosis much faster. The keto diet in turn also helps to enhance intermittent fasting. The keto diet is a carb "fast" all on its own. Fasting is easier with the absence of carbs, which will help you to overcome hunger and cravings. When you combine the two, your body will clean out waste and your body becomes more efficient. It provides even more protection against diseases such as type two diabetes and cardiovascular disease. It will also help to accelerate weight loss.

The ketogenic diet has the extra benefit in intermittent fasting that it'll help to keep your blood sugar stable. It will tend to level out during fasting periods, but if you go back to eating, your blood sugar can spike again. With the ketogenic diet, your blood sugar will stay evened out. With the ketogenic diet, you won't experience blood spikes because your body will stay in ketosis. This means that your body will continue to rely on ketones instead of glucose and having the two paired together means that you can avoid the "keto flu".

Ideally, with the ketogenic diet you'll want to use a method that allows you to fast between twelve to forty-eight hours at a time. Still, you can find what's best for you by trial and error. Remember to pay attention to your discomfort threshold. You'll need to make sure that you at the right number of calories on any of your eating windows. If you don't eat enough, then you will cause yourself metabolic issues, but too many calories will steal you away from the progress that you've made.

On the keto diet you'll need to limit various foods, especially if you're using intermittent fasting with it. Here's a general rule of thumb to follow. Don't eat any of the following.

- Anything Sugary: This includes soda, pastries, fruit juices and candy
- Grains & Grain Products: Avoid bread, pasta, rice and cereal.
- Potatoes, carrots, sweet potatoes and other starchy root vegetables
- You should avoid most fruit, but berries are allowed
- Avoid beans and legumes
- Avoid alcohol whenever possible.
- Avoid unhealthy fats such as corn oil vegetable oils, mayonnaise, etc.
- Most diet products should be avoided. Always check the label for sugar and carb content.

When you're looking for food that you can eat on the keto diet, make sure that you look on the labels to make sure that there aren't hidden sugars, unhealthy fats or carbs that will affect your ketone levels.

Some Extra Benefits

There are some extra benefits or benefits that are boosted when you combine the ketogenic diet with intermittent fasting.

- **Extra Weight Loss:** While you can't tell if you're losing more weight than you would have otherwise, you will lose weight more quickly when you combine these two diet methods. This is because your body will not come out of the state of ketosis, which turns your body into a fat burning machine by using ketones as a source of energy instead of glucose.

- **Increased Muscle Gain:** Remember that human growth hormone is produced when you use the ketogenic diet as well as when you fast, which will actually help you to gain muscle more quickly. Just make sure that you throw in some weight and resistance training as well.

- **Speedy Recovery:** If you plan to start working out more often, these two methods will help to speed up your recovery for the same reason that it promotes muscle gain. Human growth hormone will get you back on your feet faster even after a hard, grueling day of work.

- **Healthy Skin:** Humane growth hormone starts to lower naturally as you go through the aging process. However, with the ketogenic diet as well as intermittent fasting helping you to produce more, you'll see healthier more resilient skin that won't show as much sagging or wrinkles.

- **A Clear Mind:** Remember that intermittent fasting can help you to build a better brain because the state of ketosis is healthy for your brain and triggers neural pathways, which will help to improve your memory. It will also help mental clarity as well as focus.

Keto Recipes Good for Fasting

If you're going to use the ketogenic diet with intermittent fasting, then you'll want to try out these easy to use recipes!

Easy Italian Omelet

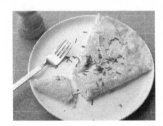

Serves: 1 **Time:** 15 Minutes

Serves: 401 **Calories:** 401 **Net Carbs:** 5.4 Grams **Protein:** 37.8 Grams **Fats:** 24.8 Grams

Ingredients:

- 2 Eggs / 2 Ounces Mozzarella
- 1 Tablespoon Water
- 1 Tablespoon Butter / 5 Slices Tomato
- 6 Basil Leaves, Fresh / 3 Slices Soppressata

Directions:

1. Mix your eggs and water together, and then add in the butter, allowing it to melt.
2. Pour your eggs in and let them sit for thirty minutes. Lay your meat onto half of the eggs, and then lay the basil, tomato and cheese on top. Sprinkle in salt and pepper.
3. Cook until your egg has set, and then fold the other half over so it covers your ingredients.
4. Put a lid on your skillet and cook for another two minutes so that your egg is cooked completely through.

Smoked Salmon with Goat Cheese

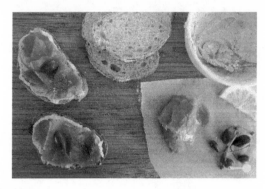

Serves: 16 **Time:** 25 Minutes

Calories: 46 **Net carbs:** 0.9 Grams **Proteins:** 3.43 Grams **Fats:** 3.33 Grams

Ingredients:

- 3.9 Ounces Radicchio
- 4 Ounces Smoked Salmon
- 2 Cloves Garlic
- Sea Salt & Black Pepper to Taste
- 1 Tablespoon Basil
- 1 Tablespoon Rosemary
- 1 Tablespoon Oregano
- 8 Ounces Goat Cheese, Softened

Directions:

1. Mince your basil, oregano and rosemary fine, and then grate your garlic. Mix your herbs, goat cheese, and garlic, salt and pepper together until it's well combined.
2. Slice the stem from your radicchio, and then take the leave apart until you have sixteen. Wash and dry your leaves, and then put a piece of salmon on each one before topping with your cheese mixture.
3. Season with pepper before chilling for at least twenty minutes before serving.

Cranberry Muffins

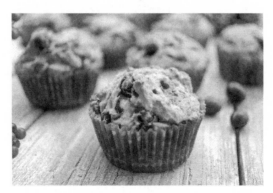

Serves: 15 **Time:** 30 Minutes

Calories: 110.7 **Protein:** 4 Grams **Net Carbs:** 5.7 Grams **Fat:** 8.2 Grams

Ingredients:

- 1 Tablespoon Vanilla
- ¼ Cup Olive Oil
- ½ Cup Vanilla Sugar Free Syrup
- 4 Eggs, Large
- ½ Cup Splenda
- ½ Teaspoon Sea Salt, Fine
- 3 Tablespoons Cinnamon
- 1 Teaspoon Nutmeg
- 1 Teaspoon Baking Powder
- 1 ¼ Cups Flaxseed Meal
- 1 Cup Cranberries, Fresh & Whole

Directions:

1. Start by preheating your oven to 350, and then butter your muffin tins.
2. Put your cranberries in a pot, and pour boiling water over them. Allow them to sit for five minutes.
3. Mix your dry and wet ingredients separately before combining them. Keep the cranberries separate for now.
4. Allow the mixture to stand for ten minutes so that it can thicken.
5. Add your cranberries in, and then spoon into your muffin tins.
6. Bake for seventeen minutes.

Almond Bread

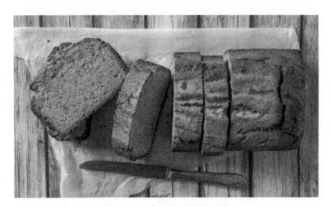

Serves: 8 **Time:** 20 Minutes

Calories: 84.1 **Net Carbs:** 2.6 Grams **Protein:** 4.3 Grams **Fat:** 6.8 Grams

Ingredients:

- ¾ Cup Almond Flour
- 1 ½ Teaspoons Baking Powder
- ¼ Teaspoon Garlic Powder
- ¼ Teaspoon Onion Powder
- ¼ Teaspoon Sea Salt, Fine
- 5 Teaspoons Butter
- 2 Eggs, Large

Directions:

1. Start by heating your oven to 375, and then mix all of your dry ingredients into a bowl.
2. Melt your butter in a microwave for a minute or until completely melted.
3. Scramble your eggs, and then mix your butter in. add in your dry ingredients, mixing well.

4. Pour the mixture into the muffin pan, and bake for fifteen minutes.

Cauliflower Casserole

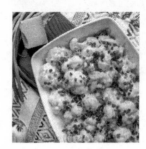

Serves: 9 **Time:** 30 Minutes

Calories: 181.8 **Net Carbs:** 5.3 Grams **Protein:** 8 Grams **Fat:** 14.9 Grams

Ingredients:

- 1 Medium Head Cauliflower, Raw
- 4 Ounces Cream Cheese / ½ Cup Sour Cream
- 4 Tablespoons Parmesan Cheese, Shredded
- 3 Sliced Hardwood Smoked Bacon
- 1 Stalk Green Onion / 1 Teaspoon Garlic Powder
- 1 Cup Cheddar Cheese, Shredded

Directions:

1. Heat your oven to 35 and then cut your cauliflower into small pieces.
2. Cook your bacon.
3. Boil your cauliflower until it's softened.
4. Mix your cream cheese, sour cream, bacon, onions, parmesan cheese, and garlic together.

5. Drain your cauliflower and place it on top of your cream cheese mixture, and mash it as if it was potatoes.

6. Get out an eight by eight inch baking dish, putting your cheddar on top, and then two slices of crushed bacon.

7. Cook for twenty minutes before serving.

Bacon & Feta Bites

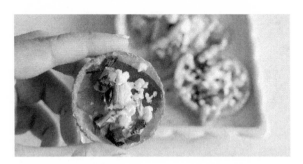

Serves: 24 **Time:** 25 Minutes

Calories: 24 **Net Carbs:** 1.08 Grams **Protein:** 3.66 Grams **Fat:** 5.74 Grams

Ingredients:

- ¼ Cup Green Onions, Chopped
- Sea Salt & Black Pepper to taste
- ¼ Cup Feta Cheese
- 8 Bacon Slices, Cooked
- 3 Tablespoons Sriracha Mayonnaise
- 2 Cups Mozzarella, Shredded
- ¾ Cup Almond Flour

Directions:

1. Heat your oven to 350 degrees.

2. Heat your skillet and then cook your almond flour and mozzarella together, stirring constantly. It should form a dough consistency within five minutes.

3. Put the dough between two pieces of parchment, rolling it out. Use a cookie cutter and make twenty-four circles.

4. Put them into a muffin in, topping with feta, bacon and onion. Bake for fifteen minutes.

5. Peel the liner off, and then top with mayo before serving.

Easy Kale Chips

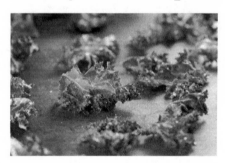

Serves: 1 **Time:** 22 Minutes

Calories: 80.5 Grams **Net Carbs:** 1.29 Grams **Protein:** 1.82 Grams **Fats:** 7.15 Grams

Ingredients:

- 1 Tablespoon Seasoned Salt
- 2 Tablespoons Olive Oil
- 1 Bunch Kale, Large & Fresh

Directions:

1. Heat your oven to 350, and then take the stems off the kale. Wash your kale leaves before drying them. Ripe the kale, putting them in a bag with oil, shaking so that the kale is well coated.

2. Put the kale on a cookie sheet before spreading it out.

3. Sprinkle with sea salt and cook for twelve minutes.

Fried Mac & Cheese

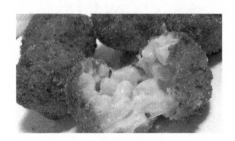

Serves: 12 **Time:** 1 Hour

Calories: 70 **Net Carbs:** 1.8 Grams **Proteins:** 4.5 Grams **Fat:** 4.71 Grams

Ingredients:

- ¾ Teaspoon Rosemary
- 2 Teaspoons Paprika
- 3 Eggs
- 1 Teaspoon Turmeric
- 1 Cauliflower Head, Riced
- 1 ½ Cups Cheddar Cheese

Directions:

1. Start my microwaving your riced cauliflower for five minute, and ring the water out.
2. Mix the eggs into your riced cauliflower, making sure it's mixed well. Then add in your cheese and spices, mixing again.
3. Form into patties and heat up some oil in a skillet.
4. Fry until browned on both sides.

Chili Cheese Muffins

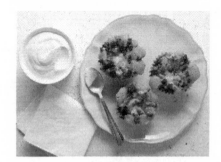

Serves: 12 **Time:** 45 Minutes

Calories: 110 **Net Carbs:** 0.5 Grams **Proteins:** 6.8 Grams **Fats:** 8.84 Grams

Ingredients:

- ½ Teaspoon Baking Soda
- 3 Eggs
- 2 Cups Cheddar Cheese, Packed
- ½ Teaspoon Sea Salt, Fine
- 1 ¼ Cups Almond Flours

Directions:

1. Set your oven to 350.
2. Combine your baking soda, flour, and salt in a food processor. Pulse until the eggs are well combined.
3. Add in your tablespoon of pepper and cheese.
4. Spoon the batter into muffin tins, and make sure that there's a quarter cup in each.
5. Sprinkle the remaining pepper on top.
6. Put it in the oven for twenty-five to thirty minutes.

A Keto & Fasting Shopping List

You can use this shopping list if you're using an intermittent diet or if you're using a ketogenic diet. Its ketogenic friendly, but it's basically the same list. However, if you choose not to pair your intermittent fasting with the ketogenic diet, you'll be allowed carbs.

Get the Right Meat

You'll want to avoid highly processed meat including some sausages, hot dogs, and even some bacon. Some lunch meat is fine, but make sure that it doesn't contain harmful additives. You'll want to focus on organic cuts and grass-fed meats whenever possible. High quality meat is better for your body. You'll find a list below.

- Steak
- Prime Rib
- Roast Beef
- Veal
- Baby Back Ribs
- Ground Beef
- Corned Beef
- Hamburger
- Stew Meats
- Heart
- Liver
- Tongue
- Kidney Offal
- Bison

- Lamb
- Goat
- Most Fish (Including Tuna, Salmon, Catfish, Trout, Mackerel, Halibut, Mahi-Mahi, Crab, Lobster, mussels, Scallops, Shrimp, Cod, Bas, Orange Roughy, Tilapia and Haddock
- Most Poultry including Duck, chicken, Quail, Turkey, Wild Game, Chicken Broth, Turkey Bacon, Cornish Hens, Turkey Sausage, Eggs
- All Pork including Ground Pork, Bacon, Ham, Pork Chops, Tenderloin and Pork Rinds

Dairy Products

There are some dairy products that you should avoid such as reduced fat or low-fat dairy products. You should also avoid fermented products such as yogurt or kefir. Avoid dairy products that are high in sugar or have added fruit. You should also avoid milk, even whole milk, evaporated, half condensed milk as well as half and half. Just remember that even when you indulge in the dairy products that you can have, you should make sure that they don't make up a large majority of your calories.

- Full Fat Greek Yogurt
- Heavy Creams
- Sour Cream
- Butter, Grass Fed
- Mayonnaise
- Ghee
- Heavy Whipping Cream

- Cheeses including Ricotta, String, Cream, Cottage Cheese, Goat, Blue Cheese, Colby, Mozzarella, Brie, Cheddar, Swiss, Parmesan, Feta & Monterrey Jack

Oils & Fats

Fats will make up the bulk of your calories if you're using the ketogenic diet, which will help when you're using intermittent fasting as well. You'll just need a few more items from the grocery store such as grass-fed butter or coconut oil, which are excellent choices. You can also use oils such as extra virgin olive oil to make homemade dressings. You should reserve seeds and nuts for snacks only, and you should limit them even when using the intermittent fasting lifestyle, they're high in carbs, so they'll actually slow down your weight loss. You should avoid hydrogenated or partially hydrogenated oils that are found in margarines and fast food. Avocado oil or MCT oil are also an option.

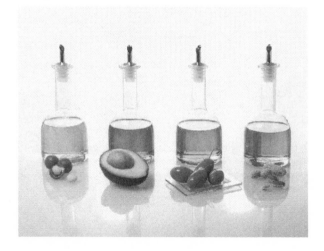

Nuts

If you really want nuts, go for almonds or almond butter, hazelnuts, macadamias, sesame seeds, chia seeds, pumpkin seeds, walnuts, pistachios, pecans, or sunflower seeds.

Vegetables

Don't forget that vegetables are important to any diet! When working with the ketogenic diet. Vegetables should make up the majority of what you buy. You should concentrate on leafy greens since they contain very few carbs and are packed with minerals and vitamins. You should avoid certain vegetables if you're using the ketogenic diet including starchy vegetables such as parsnips, sweet potatoes, potatoes, carrots and corns. You should avoid some types of squash, including summer squash which are high in carbs. Below you'll find some vegetables that you can buy for both the ketogenic diet and intermittent fasting.

- Radicchio
- Iceberg Lettuce
- Romaine Lettuce
- Swiss Chard
- Spinach
- Bok Choy
- Kale
- Leafy Greens
- Bean Sprouts
- Artichoke Hearts
- Green Beans
- Brussel Sprouts

- Garlic
- Broccoli
- Bell Pepper
- Onions
- Asparagus
- Celery
- Cucumber
- White Mushrooms
- Portobello Mushrooms
- Green Olives
- Black Olives
- Spaghetti Squash
- Snow Peas
- Zucchini
- Okra
- Snow Peas
- Leeks
- Cauliflower
- Cabbage
- Artichokes

Fruit

On the ketogenic diet fruit should only be consumed in moderation, but if you're just using intermittent fasting, then you can eat a lot more fruits. Use fruits as a treat so that you don't spike your blood sugar levels. On the ketogenic diet you'll need to avoid most fruit because it's high in sugar and high in carbs. You should avoid fruits such as mangos, watermelon, pears, oranges, apples and bananas. You should also avoid fruit juice and dried fruit. Below you'll find the fruits that you can enjoy on the ketogenic diet, especially when using intermittent fasting.

- Avocados
- Cranberries
- Cherries
- Raspberries
- Strawberries
- Blueberries
- Mulberries

Herbs & Spices

You can use almost any herbs and spices so long as they don't have hidden carbs and sugars, which is why you should avoid spice blends when possible. However, fresh herbs are often better because they provide your body with more essential nutrients and minerals.

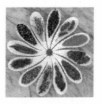

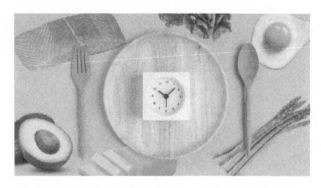

Should You Use Both?

You already know that you should contact your doctor if you want to use intermittent fasting, and if you want to start a drastic overhaul such as the ketogenic diet, you'll need to talk to your doctor as well. It goes without saying that if you wish to do both, your health care professional should be notified. The will be some cases where you shouldn't use either. If you have a serious health problem such as cardiovascular disease, then you'll likely not want to go too long without food since it can cause heart palpitations. Pregnant or nursing women are not recommended to use intermittent fasting along with the ketogenic diet. While intermittent fasting and the ketogenic diet have both been proven to be helpful with cancer patients, it is not recommended to use both diets together when going through stressful processes such as chemotherapy. The bottom line is, you should always talk to your doctor to see if either of these diet methods are for you. If you are taking medication that needs to be taken with food, then intermittent fasting may not be for you either.

Made in the USA
San Bernardino, CA
10 December 2018